MYOFASCIAL STRETCHING

A Guide to Self-Treatment

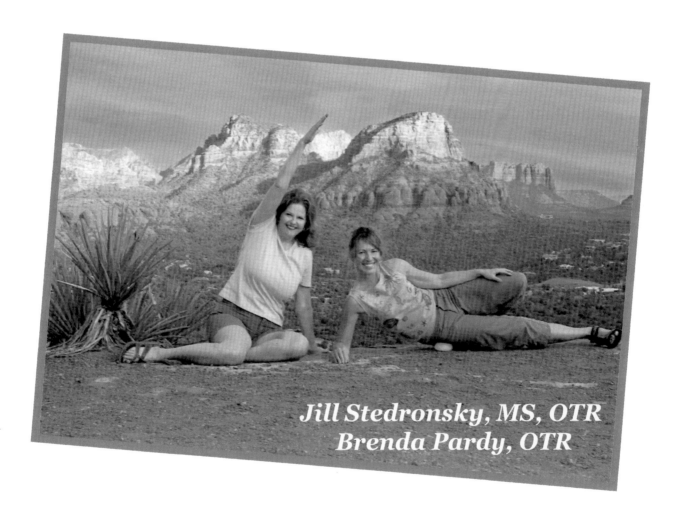

Jill Stedronsky, MS, OTR
Brenda Pardy, OTR

Foreword by
John F. Barnes, PT

DISCLAIMER

Not all of the stretches outlined in this book are appropriate for every person. These stretches should be utilized consistent with common sense and your physical or other limitations, under the supervision of your therapist or doctor. This book is not intended to replace advice from a qualified medical practitioner. Seek a medical opinion if you have any concerns about your health and whether these stretches are appropriate for your conditions. The authors do not accept any liability whatsoever for injuries resulting from failure to follow this advice.

The authors and their agents shall not be liable in the event of damages of any sort, including incidental or consequential damages, in connection with, or arising out of the furnishing, performance or use of the stretches, the balls, associated instructions and/or claims of benefit.

The authors of the book have used their best efforts in preparing the stretches and descriptions. The authors and their agents make no warranty of any kind, expressed or implied, with regard to the stretches or the documentation contained in this book.

Aardvark Global Publishing Company, LLC
Denver Myofascial Release
6535 South Dayton Street
Suite 3800
Greenwood Village, CO 80111

Cover design by Justin and Brenda Pardy
Cover photo by Maria Liliana Perez
Cover photo digitally enhanced by Herrera Photography
Photo taken at Airport Mesa, Sedona, AZ

ISBN: 1-4276-0216-6

Copyright © 2006 Jill Stedronsky & Brenda J. Pardy,
Second Edition Copyright © 2008
Denver, Colorado

All rights reserved. This book may not be duplicated in any way without the expressed written consent of the authors. The information contained herein is for the personal use of the reader, and may not be incorporated in any commercial program, other books or any kind of software without written consent. Making copies of this book or any portion of it for any purpose is a violation of the United States copyright laws.

DEDICATION

To John F. Barnes, PT,
our teacher and mentor,
developer of John F. Barnes Myofascial Release.
You have transformed our lives and the lives of our patients.
Thank you for being a Renegade,
for boldly going where few have dared to go.

ACKNOWLEDGMENTS

To all the wonderful Myofascial Release Therapists at
Therapy on the Rocks and throughout the world
who have crossed our paths and shared
in the adventure.

To the many patients who have been some of our best teachers.

To Tina Matsuoka, MPT, amazing therapist at Therapy on the Rocks,
who first taught us Myofascial Stretching.

To Jo Klein, for her hours and hours of dedicated editorial work
resulting in a much more user-friendly book.

To Justin Pardy, for his invaluable computer expertise, assistance and patience.

To Sandy Do, PT, for her incredible expertise and unwavering support
through Jill's healing journey.

To Lisa Ganfield, OTR, for mentoring Jill
and providing her with an opportunity to work in an MFR clinic.

To Jody Hendryx, PT, RMT, for being there for Jill
at all the right times in all the right ways.

To Pete Morton, PhD, for his love, support,
and the invaluable life lessons.

To Bill Pardy,
who tolerated his home being dismantled for a photography studio,
his kitchen taken over for an editing room
and weekend plans disrupted by deadlines.

To our families, for their constant love and support.

FOREWORD

Self-treatment is a powerful way for patients to enhance their progress while receiving Myofascial Release (MFR) Therapy. After all, it was through exploration in treating my own back pain that I began to develop the MFR paradigm. In my Myofascial Release Seminars and Myofascial Release Treatment Centers, we teach self-treatment and encourage therapists and patients alike to take responsibility for their own healing. While our Myofascial Release Treatment Centers have developed handouts of individual stretches, until now there has not been a collection of self-treatment techniques in book form. It is exciting to see this project come to fruition.

Jill and Brenda are extraordinary therapists of the highest caliber and have done an excellent job capturing the essence of MFR principles and presenting the stretches with clear photographs and concise explanations. I envision therapists offering the Myofascial Stretching book to clients as an important part of their home programs. In addition, people with limited access to an MFR therapist now have a valuable resource guide to advance their own healing.

It is always a pleasure for a teacher to see his students grow and evolve. I am very proud of Jill and Brenda for their accomplishments and I highly endorse this book for anyone seeking the authentic healing that Myofascial Release has to offer.

John F. Barnes, PT
Myofascial Release Treatment Centers and Seminars

JILL'S STORY

I lived with chronic pain throughout my body for 20 years as a result of multiple traumas suffered as a child and young adult. Before discovering John F. Barnes Myofascial Release (MFR), I had been diagnosed with chronic fatigue syndrome, fibromyalgia, depression and numerous orthopedic conditions. Chiropractic, traditional physical and occupational therapy, acupuncture and massage provided temporary relief. As an Occupational Therapist with many resources at my disposal, healing remained elusive. I tried many modalities including Pilates, yoga and weight training. Despite high caliber instructors, my pain got worse because of the severe fascial restrictions pulling me out of alignment. I was eventually forced to give up the activities I loved, including telemark skiing, hiking and biking. I could barely hold down a part time job and even walking was painful. Two surgeons told me I'd never ski again without bilateral knee surgery. Shoulder and ankle operations were also recommended. Other doctors proposed antidepressants and pain killers. I refused all surgeries and medications, believing there was another answer.

I had been exposed to Myofascial Release as an OT student, but it wasn't until hitting the proverbial "rock bottom" that I finally found an MFR therapist in Denver. My body immediately responded and knew this was what it needed. I traveled to John Barnes' clinic in Sedona, Arizona to undergo two weeks of intensive therapy. In addition to receiving excellent treatment, I was introduced to the concept of treating myself and the principles of Myofascial Stretching. Returning home with less pain than I'd had in years, I continued to receive therapy and began taking MFR Seminars. A tremendous amount of my energy went into Myofascial Stretching. Hours were spent alone tuning into my body discovering where my fascial restrictions were and how to release them. I experimented with techniques learned in Sedona, and intuitively started to develop my own. Upon learning to feel the releases, Myofascial Stretching became a part of my lifestyle as I gratefully returned to previous activities. I could now release tight tissue while watching a movie, riding in the car or on my bike, dancing at a concert and engaging in conversation at a party. Props such as trees and logs, chairlift supports, doorways, rocks, benches and picnic tables helped me to engage and release fascial restrictions. I stretched while talking on the phone, waiting in line, typing at the computer and even sitting on the toilet. Increased body awareness, greater focus, presence and ability to concentrate on two things at once were unexpected and welcomed benefits of this process.

As my body continued to untwist, unwind and free itself of the 'Myofascial Straightjacket' in which it had been imprisoned, other modalities became more helpful. Spinal manipulations would now hold. Weak muscles previously encased in tight fascia could finally activate and become strong. I found that MFR can be the missing link and exponentially increase the effectiveness of Chiropractic, traditional PT and OT, acupuncture, massage, Pilates, yoga and weight training for people with major fascial restrictions.

Today, I have returned to pursuing the activities I love. I am blessed with a successful Myofascial Release Practice and teach all my clients Myofascial Stretching. My body is strong, healthy, virtually pain free and supports me in amazing ways. I am a more grounded, centered, intuitive person as a result of tuning into and listening to my body. I live in a constant state of gratitude. My intention is to offer this story and these techniques to anyone else in pain that might benefit from my experience. Like anything in life, you get out of it what you put into it. Myofascial Stretching is not a quick fix. It is a Journey. It takes time for a body to become tight and twisted. It takes time and awareness for it to release and realign.

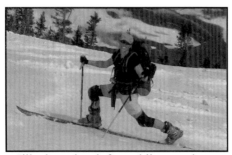

Jill takes a break from skiing to release the front of her hip.

Enjoy!

Jill Stedronsky, MS, OTR

BRENDA'S STORY

As an Occupational Therapist of fifteen years, I knew all about using good body mechanics. Despite this knowledge, I injured my back while lifting a heavy tote bag from an awkward angle. The next morning, I stood up and passed out from the pain of a bulging disc. I was sent home from the ER on painkillers and muscle relaxants for two weeks of bed rest. I began physical therapy three times per week, tapering off when I returned to work six weeks after my injury. I was discharged to a rigorous home exercise program after three months of traditional PT. Six months later I was quite pleased to be pain-free and able to move smoothly in all directions. I had expected to have back pain forever. The total cost of this injury including medical bills and lost wages was about $10,000.

I had been receiving fliers from John F. Barnes Myofascial Release Treatment Centers and Seminars. When the Pediatric Course came to Cheyenne, Wyoming I signed up. I practiced the techniques on friends and family members young and old with fabulous results, then began to integrate Myofascial Release into treatment sessions. My clients progressed more rapidly and maintained their gains more easily when MFR was part of their program. Needless to say, I signed up for more and more courses.

When Jill Stedronsky and I crossed paths we began meeting weekly to trade treatments, study and consult. Jill helped me build my repertoire of self-treatment ideas. Then the inevitable happened. Toward the end of a fantastic day of downhill skiing with my husband, I fell on a steep, narrow run. I had to force my way up from a twisted position. As we drove home, the familiar twinges of back pain from fourteen years earlier returned. I stretched that night, but the next morning couldn't get out of bed. In a panic I called my colleague, mentor and friend Jill. She talked me through a Myofascial Stretching protocol while flat on my back. By noon I was moving slowly. After three treatment sessions with Jill and spending many hours stretching and using the inflated balls as described in this book, I recovered in less than a week without missing a day of work. There was an enormous savings in time and cost compared to my first injury. I was happy to escape the impact of living through months of pain, suffering and loss of function.

Always a proponent of home activities for my clients, my own experience of Myofascial Stretching took the academic concept to a much deeper level of understanding. I began in earnest to teach both adults and children how to release their own fascial restrictions, giving hand written instructions with my most artistic stick figures. One day Jill mentioned her desire to compile all the stretches she had learned, ones she developed herself and those I created into a usable format for our patients. I offered to collaborate on the project. The result is this book, which provides over 130 photographed Myofascial Stretching techniques to assist you in releasing your own fascial restrictions to achieve better health, alignment and function. You may not have to live with unceasing pain. I don't. I'm glad you've decided to give Myofascial Stretching a try.

Blessings!

Brenda Pardy, OTR

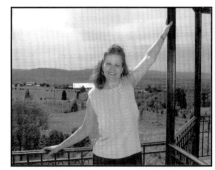

In the midst of entertaining guests on her deck
Brenda takes a break to release her shoulder.

INDICATIONS

Some of the most common conditions for which Myofascial Stretching is appropriate are:

Auto Injuries
Back Pain
Carpal Tunnel Syndrome
Chronic Fatigue Syndrome
Elbow, Wrist and Hand Pain
Fibromyalgia
Headaches
Hip Pain
Jaw Pain, TMJ Dysfunction
Knee, Ankle and Foot Pain
Migraines
Myofascial Pain Syndrome
Neck Pain
Osteoarthritis
Plantar Fascitis
Restriction in Motion
Scarring and Adhesions
Sciatica
Scoliosis
Shoulder Pain
Sports Injuries
Stress and Tension Related Problems
Thoracic Outlet Syndrome
Whiplash
Women's Health Issues
Work Injuries

CONTRAINDICATIONS

***Some Myofascial Stretching techniques
may not be appropriate
for people with the following conditions:***

Acute Rheumatoid Arthritis
Advanced Diabetes
Aneurysm
Anticoagulant Therapy Treatment
Healing Fracture
Hematoma
Joint Instability
Malignancy
Open Wound
Osteoporosis
Swelling
Systemic or Localized Infection

Acute Disc Problem
Consult a doctor or therapist for most appropriate techniques.

Pregnancy
Avoid 4-1, 4-4, 7-2, 8-1 thru 8-5, 12-1 thru 12-3.
Be gentle with all other techniques, especially in later stages of pregnancy.

Spondylolisthesis and Spinal Stenosis
Be cautious with low back hyperextension especially 12-2 and 12-3.

***Please seek a medical opinion
before beginning this or any exercise program.
Talk to your health care provider about
any concerns you may have.***

Extremely Important

It is essential to read the Introduction, FAQs and Instructions
to gain maximum benefit from Myofascial Stretching.
After completing a few techniques
please re-read to integrate the concepts more thoroughly.

Be sure to work on both sides of the body
even if pain is only on one side.

TABLE OF CONTENTS

Disclaimer	*ii*
Dedication	*iii*
Acknowledgments	*iv*
Foreword	*v*
Jill's Story	*vi*
Brenda's Story	*vii*
Indications	*viii*
Contraindications	*ix*
Extremely Important	*x & 11*

Introduction	2

Frequently Asked Questions (FAQs)	3
What Is Fascia and Why Is It Important?	3
What Is a Fascial Restriction and How Does It Occur?	3
What Is Myofascial Release?	3
How Does Myofascial Stretching Differ From Traditional Stretching?	3
What Does a Release Feel Like?	4
Can I Hurt Myself With Myofascial Stretching?	4

Instructions	6
Getting Ready	6
Deciding Where to Begin	6
Continuing On	6
Planning Your Session	7
Tools	7
How to Use the Inflatable Balls	8
How to Do Myofascial Stretching With Active Elongation	8
And Finally . . .	9
References	9

Myofascial Stretching Guide	10

Section 1 - Neck & Jaw	12
Section 2 - Shoulder	15
Section 3 - Upper Extremity *(arm, elbow, forearm, wrist, hand)*	22
Section 4 - Lateral Trunk	26
Section 5 - Spine	27
Section 6 - Upper & Mid Back	28
Section 7 - Low Back	30
Section 8 - Abdomen &Front of Hip	32
Section 9 - Hips & Buttocks	36
Section 10 - Upper Leg	38
Section 11 - Lower Leg	42
Section 12 - Multiple Release Techniques	47

About the Authors	50
Testimonials	51
Ordering and Contact Information	52
Order Form	53

INTRODUCTION

Myofascial Stretching is a self-treatment technique that results in permanent lengthening of the body's connective tissue and has the capacity to dramatically improve health and quality of life. It follows the principles of Myofascial Release (MFR), utilizing sustained pressure and active elongation into restrictions in the fascial system. Many of the techniques were developed by the authors while engaging in self-treatment or working with clients. Some are taught at the Myofascial Release Treatment Centers in Sedona, AZ and Paoli, PA. Others stretches may seem familiar to you, but are performed with Myofascial Release principles in mind. Two ways to do Myofascial Stretching are included: one uses a small inflatable ball and the other one utilizes active elongation of the muscles. These two methods complement each other. It can be very effective to first release an area of tightness with the ball and then follow up with an active stretch to that same region.

The book is divided into twelve sections relating to different parts of the body. This arbitrary division is for simplification in organizing the information. In treatment the body is always considered as a whole. Read the instructions to help you decide where to start. If you are still unsure of how to proceed, go to the chart on page 10 for ideas of which techniques may be related to your problem area.

While there is a narrative description along with each photograph, it is *IMPERATIVE* the reader study the information for releasing the fascial system described in the Frequently Asked Questions and Instructions. This stretching protocol will likely be very different from anything you have learned before. If done properly, it will result in permanent release of the fascial system, rather than temporary gains obtained through traditional stretching.

This book was written for the lay person who has chronic pain, muscular tightness or postural dysfunction. It was also designed for doctors and therapists to prescribe home exercise programs for their patients (and themselves!!!). When used alone this book can be a valuable resource for healing chronic pain. We would like to stress the benefit of receiving MFR Therapy from a skilled practitioner in order to experience the feel of the fascial system, to address areas that are difficult to release on your own and to receive insights and guidance into your particular condition. Myofascial Stretching also works well in conjunction with other forms of treatment you may already be receiving, greatly enhancing their effectiveness. When fascial restrictions are identified and released, quantum leaps in healing can be achieved.

FREQUENTLY ASKED QUESTIONS (FAQs)

What Is Fascia and Why Is It Important?

Fascia is the tough connective tissue surrounding every cell from head to toe like a three-dimensional spider web. It provides support and flexibility to all structures of the body. Modern medicine tends to look at muscles, bones and organs in isolation, generally ignoring the importance of the global system that connects it all together. Releasing restrictions in the fascia can be the missing link in resolving problematic cases of pain and dysfunction.

What Is a Fascial Restriction and How Does It Occur?

A fascial restriction is a thickening, shortening or tightening in the connective tissue caused by injury, trauma, inflammation or poor posture. Restrictions can adhere to and put abnormal pressure on nerves, muscles, blood vessels, bones, organs and the brain, resulting in inefficient function of these structures. Pain, limitation of motion and structural misalignment are some of the consequences.

What Is Myofascial Release?

Myofascial Release, as developed and taught by John F. Barnes, PT, is a gentle, hands on approach used to free up fascial restrictions throughout the body. The therapist releases the tight fascia by applying sustained pressure into the fascial barrier or restriction, allowing permanent elongation of the tissues. As fascial layers are released, the client gains greater flexibility. This results in decreased pain, enhanced daily functional abilities, refined athletic performance, increased ease of movement and improved structural balance and integrity.

How Does Myofascial Stretching Differ From Traditional Stretching?

There are four primary ways that Myofascial Stretching differs from traditional stretching. The first one involves the time element. All Myofascial Stretches, with or without the ball, must be held continuously for a minimum of 90 to 120 seconds before the fascia even begins to let go. When held three to five minutes, additional releases may occur. *THE TIME ELEMENT IS CRITICAL.* Holding the stretch allows a release of not only the elastic and muscular components of the connective tissue, but the collagenous component as well. Traditional 30 second stretching only affects the elastic and muscular portions, providing temporary results.

The second way Myofascial Stretching differs from traditional passive stretching is the concept of active elongation. Active elongation is what allows one to engage the fascial barrier. For example, extend your arm out to the side with your wrist bent backwards. Feel a stretch. Now, in the same position, REACH, TELESCOPE, or ELONGATE your arm as if you are trying to make it longer. Feel how that engages the tissue along the entire length of your arm into your hand. The fascial barrier is the point at which you feel resistance to the stretch.

The third essential difference is the need to be consciously present throughout the process of Myofascial Stretching. It is exponentially more effective when you are able to focus on the tension in the tissue, direct your breath into the restriction, notice the resulting slack as the release takes place, elongate into the next barrier and wait for another release to occur. Regular practice of these techniques with conscious attention to what you are feeling and to your breath will increase body awareness, patience and intuition. Myofascial Stretching can become a form of body-centered meditation, transforming you into a more focused, centered and grounded person.

The fourth distinction is that stretching and strengthening occur simultaneously. During active elongation, muscle groups opposing the tight fascia have to contract in a sustained manner. This prolonged isometric contraction of muscles against the resistance of the fascial barrier strengthens them, helping to maintain the elongated state of the tissue you have just released.

What Does a Release Feel Like?

A release may feel like taffy lengthening or butter melting. There may be a burning or ripping sensation, pulsing, tingling or a release of heat. Sometimes there is an increase in tension followed by a sense of slack. The sensations often intensify as the release is occurring and then decrease or disappear when it is complete. You may feel the fascia connecting into other areas. This is your body talking to you. This 'fascial voice' lets you know there is a relationship between the restriction you are treating and the part of your body to which sensation is referred. Both areas need to be treated.

Some individuals feel the releases right away; for others it takes a little longer. Tune in and allow yourself to be present. Over time, with practice, you will feel the fascia let go. Until you do, know that if you maintain the stretch at the fascial barrier for at least 90 to 120 seconds, a release will probably occur whether you feel it or not.

Can I Hurt Myself With Myofascial Stretching?

No. As long as the guidelines in this book are followed you will not hurt yourself with Myofascial Stretching. It is impossible to force the fascial system to let go. Rather, one must wait patiently at each barrier for it to release. Before beginning this program, consult the contraindications list. Please seek a qualified medical opinion if you have one of the conditions on the list or have questions and concerns about your body's response to the stretches. Always use common sense.

While performing a technique, your symptoms may be reproduced. If so, do not be alarmed. You are probably treating the cause of your pain. Myofascial Stretching can be uncomfortable. If necessary, back off on the intensity to a more tolerable level. However, if your gut instinct says this technique is harmful to you, then stop immediately. Individuals who are frail and/or elderly should exercise caution and start out with a softer (less inflated) ball. In addition, one should always be careful when using a ball around sensitive areas such as the xiphoid process at the base of the breastbone and the last two 'floating' ribs located at the bottom of the ribcage on the back and side of the trunk just above the waist.

There are times when an individual may feel emotions connected with a fascial restriction or release. This can happen because a memory related to the current pain was triggered or trapped energy from a previous trauma was accessed. It can also occur without situational context. You may feel like crying or your body may want to shake or move. If this should happen, stay present with what you are feeling and breathe into the emotions and sensations. Allow yourself to cry, shake, move or vocalize. These feelings are coming up for a reason. Healing occurs more readily when we allow ourselves to feel our emotions. Trapped inside of us and unexpressed, they can materialize as pain and dysfunction. This is a powerful example of the mind/body connection. With the emotional energy discharged, complete healing can now take place. If you would like support in dealing with emotions that may surface with the physical releases, contact a therapist[1] who has been trained to assist in this process.

---

[1] Visit www.myofascialrelease.com for a directory of therapists.

INSTRUCTIONS

Getting Ready:

Set time aside to be alone without interruption. Create a setting that encourages you to focus. Some people light candles and play music. Others prefer silence. Find what works best for you.

Deciding Where to Begin:

Tune into your body and become aware of sensations of tightness and pain. Browse through the book and find a technique that seems to be related to your particular ailment. The authors have found that releasing an area of tightness with the ball and then following up with an active stretch to that same region can be extremely effective. However, there are places on the body where it is difficult to use a ball, so an elongation stretch is the best option. Listen to what your body needs and start experimenting. There are no wrong choices. Pick a technique and go for it.

Continuing On:

While treating your symptomatic area, you may find your attention being drawn to sensations elsewhere. Don't be surprised if you feel a connection far removed from where you are working. If so, follow the fascial voice and focus there next. Conversely, you may feel a direct link to your pain while treating at a site distant from your symptoms. If you find that any technique feels connected to or reproduces your symptoms, stay with it and allow the release to complete. You may be on the cusp of a breakthrough. Because the fascia is one continuous web which runs head to toe, everything in the body is connected via this system. Shoulder problems may come from neck tightness and imbalance. Jaw pain can be related to restriction at the throat, front of the neck and chest, or to a rotated pelvis. Back pain is often caused by shortened tissue in the abdomen, thighs or front of the hips. Headaches can result from a restricted tailbone. Knee and foot problems may be a consequence of tightness at the hip or pelvis. Pain on one side of the body is often related to fascial restrictions on the other.

If you don't feel your attention being drawn elsewhere, continue to work near the site of pain or tightness. Be sure to treat all sides of a problem area (above/below, front/back, left/right) even if the symptoms are localized. It is very important to not get locked into the mentality of treating only where it hurts. As John Barnes says in his seminars, "Find the pain and look elsewhere for the cause."

While Myofascial Stretching does result in permanent lengthening of the connective tissue, you may notice that an area you have treated continues to tighten between sessions, refuses to release at all, or that new symptoms develop. This can be due to related fascial restrictions not yet identified. Hence, it is important to find and address all restrictions that may be contributing to the problem. If you are having difficulty knowing how to proceed, try the following. 1) Pay closer attention to the fascial voice and use your intuition. 2) Ask yourself if you have treated all sides of the problem area as described above. 3) Go to the chart on Page 10 for ideas of other techniques that may be related. If unsure of how to get started, or if running into a plateau with your particular condition, consult an MFR therapist to customize a treatment program to your individual needs.

Incomplete results may also occur if you have not developed the muscular control or core stability to support your newly acquired range of motion. The body has wisdom of its own. There are times when a restriction will not even begin to release, or that release will not be sustained, until the body has confidence that there is adequate support. This topic is beyond the scope of this book, but please be sure to work on motor control and core stability concurrently with Myofascial Stretching. Consult a therapist, doctor or trainer who specializes in this area of expertise if you have questions.

Eventually it will be beneficial to do all the techniques in the book, except ones that may be contraindicated for your specific condition. Even if you are not in pain, these techniques can improve circulation, flexibility, posture, energy flow and functional or athletic performance.

Planning Your Session:

Keep in mind it is better to go deeply into a few techniques in one session, than to race through many quickly. Quality is more important than quantity. If you only have five minutes, do one or two stretches. If you have more time, you may release one or two barriers at multiple sites, moving from one restriction to another as your attention is drawn to each. Or you may end up spending half an hour or more treating a single area to access deeper layers of a restriction. Whether you do one technique or many in any given session is up to you. Listen to your body and it will tell you what it needs.

Tools:

The four-inch ball sold with this book is a simple, inexpensive and amazing tool. It is effective for lengthening tissue and relieving pain, tightness, trigger points and muscle spasms. We have found this particular ball to have the most versatility and to be universally effective just about anywhere on the body. It can be re-inflated with a pump when it starts to lose air. Be sure to moisten the needle when re-inflating the ball. Don't force the needle into the valve as this may break the seal so that the ball will not hold air. Adjust the angle of the needle and reinsert. Softer balls found elsewhere are not as effective as this ball.

The first edition of this book referred only to the four-inch ball, which is still our favorite and considered the workhorse of Myofascial Stretching. However, we have been researching other sizes and now offer balls in three and five-inch diameters. The smaller ones have proven effective when higher intensity in a specific location is needed, when seated in a car or airplane and with children/petite adults. The larger balls can engage deeper layers of restriction in the abdomen, and spine. They can be more effective overall with larger framed adults. We recommend trying these different sized balls in various restrictions and positions to see which works best. Tennis or golf balls, rollers, pillows, large therapy balls and other tools can also be used following MFR principles if they evoke a better response in a particular area of the body. These and other tools will be addressed more specifically in our second book, with the working title of *Advanced Myofascial Stretching: Beyond the Yellow Ball.*

How to Use the Inflatable Balls:

Place the ball under an area of pain or tightness and slowly roll on it to find the point of greatest intensity. Don't roll too fast, or you may pass right over a key spot. It may take ten seconds or more to sink in deeply enough to realize you are in a restriction. When you find an area that feels hot, hard, tender, tight or refers pain/sensation to another area, stay there and allow your body to sink further into the ball. Breathe into whatever you are experiencing and continue to allow your body to soften and relax around the ball. Remain in each area for a minimum of 90 to 120 seconds, or until you feel a release. You may want to stay there longer if it feels beneficial, until the sensation you are experiencing diminishes or disappears. This allows you to access multiple layers of the fascial system. It is not uncommon to spend three to five minutes on one technique.

Because fascial restrictions are comprised of multiple barriers, each one needs to be released in order to restore full freedom of motion. When one area feels complete, roll around and seek out the next point of restriction, tenderness or tightness. Roll slowly and stay present, as the next layer may be only millimeters away from where you were just working. Sometimes a slight weight shift or change in position is all it takes to access the next layer without rolling at all. You might spend an entire session working intensively in one area, i.e. the outside of the thigh. Other times you may want to move to another body part where sensation was referred or seems to be connected in some way. Listen to what your body is telling you and allow your intuition to guide you. There is no right or wrong way to do Myofascial Stretching as long as you are following the general principles.

While lying, sitting or leaning on the ball, you may need to adapt your position to change the intensity of what you are feeling. Increase the intensity to go deeper into the restriction or to follow the tissue to the next layer as it releases. If the intensity feels too severe, decrease it to a level you can maintain for a minimum of 90 to 120 seconds. To accomplish these changes shift your weight, bend your knees, reach your arms overhead, come up on your elbows, elongate or stretch your arms, legs or torso. The force can also be modified by working on a harder or softer surface; the floor vs. a bed. The ball can be further inflated to make it harder or deflated to make it softer. Placing a hard cover book underneath the ball will raise it up and increase the amount of pressure provided. If pressure at the point of greatest intensity is too much to handle, move the ball slightly off center and circle around the painful point waiting for a release each time you move the ball. Eventually direct pressure will be tolerable. Another way to change the intensity is to use two balls simultaneously, i.e. on either side of the spine or sacrum.

How to Do Myofascial Stretching With Active Elongation:

Choose one of the stretches from the book that seems to be related to your symptoms or choose an area you have just released using the ball. Enter into the stretch slowly and consciously. When you begin to encounter a restriction, engage it further by actively telescoping that body part. Keep the intensity mild to moderate, never forcing the tissue. More is not always better. Stay present with what you are feeling. Breathe deeply, imagining the breath flowing into areas of pain and restriction. Relax and allow your body to soften while maintaining tension at the fascial barrier.

Hold every stretch for at least 90 to 120 seconds or until the intensity diminishes or disappears. At that point, alter your position slightly or elongate further to access the next layer of restriction. Now hold for an additional 90 to 120 seconds or until the fascia softens and lengthens again. Remember, there are always multiple barriers. It is important to follow the tissue as it releases into each subsequent restriction. The longer you work in an area, the more progress you can make in a single session. If sensation is referred to another part of your body, you may choose to treat there next or in a future session.

And Finally . . .

It is crucial to set aside time to practice Myofascial Stretching on a regular basis if you want to meet your goals of eliminating pain and improving health. Once your body awareness and perception of the fascial releases has heightened, you can also take advantage of opportunities to engage in Myofascial Stretching throughout your day. At work, play and home, make Myofascial Stretching a part of your routine. Think of techniques that are practical within the parameters of your environment. Follow the principles outlined in this book and look for tools or props you can use. Doorway stretches can easily be done in the office while talking to a co-worker. They can be adapted in many ways: use a tree at the park or the uprights on a chairlift. Put the ball behind your back while seated at your desk or riding in a car. Stretch your neck while talking on the phone. Place your foot on a bench at a party and release the front of your hip. As long as you keep your focus on maintaining tension at the fascial barrier, you will sense the releases while you read, peel potatoes, watch TV or work on a computer.

Use this book as a starting point. The techniques presented are simply guidelines. Tune in and discover the fascial restrictions in your body. We all have them. As you learn to identify yours and experience how it feels as they release, you will be able to use the principles described here to invent your own stretches. While treating, let go of your expectations. Tap into your creativity. Activate your imagination and explore. See where the fascial voice takes you. Where is your body asking to be released?

References
Barnes, John F., Myofascial Release, The Search for Excellence. Rehabilitation Services, Inc., Pennsylvania. 1990.

Barnes, John F., Healing Ancient Wounds, The Renegade's Wisdom. Rehabilitation Services, Inc., Pennsylvania. 2000.

MYOFASCIAL STRETCHING GUIDE

Because of the global nature of the fascial system, Myofascial Stretching does not use protocols or recipes for specific dysfunctions. Your body will benefit from all the exercises. This chart is intended to help you find those techniques which may have the most value for you.

If You Have:	*Try the Following Sections:*
Carpal Tunnel Syndrome, Elbow, Wrist, Hand Pain	1, 2, 3, 4, 5, 6, 12
Chronic Fatigue Syndrome, Fibromyalgia, Myofascial Pain	1, 2, 3, 4, 5, 6, 7, 8, 9, 10, 11, 12
Foot/Ankle Pain/Plantar Fascitis	8, 9, 10, 11
Headaches	1, 2, 3, 5, 6
Hip Pain	4, 5, 7, 8, 9, 10, 11, 12
Jaw Tension/TMJ Dysfunction	1, 5
Knee Pain	8, 9, 10, 11
Low Back Pain	4, 5, 6, 7, 8, 9, 10, 11, 12
Neck Pain	1, 2, 3, 5, 6
Sciatica	4, 5, 7, 8, 9, 10, 11, 12
Scoliosis	1, 2, 4, 5, 6, 7, 8, 9, 10, 12
Shoulder Pain	1, 2, 3, 4, 5, 6, 12
Stress/Tension Related Problems	1, 2, 3, 4, 5, 6, 7, 8, 9, 10, 11, 12
Thoracic Outlet Syndrome	1, 2, 3, 4, 5, 6, 12
Upper/Mid Back Pain	1, 2, 4, 5, 6, 12
Women's Health Issues/Pelvic Pain/Pelvic Floor Dysfunction	4, 5, 7, 8, 9, 10, 12

Extremely Important

It is essential to read the Introduction, FAQs and Instructions
to gain maximum benefit from Myofascial Stretching.
After completing a few techniques,
please re-read to integrate the concepts more thoroughly.

Be sure to work on both sides of the body
even if pain is only on one side.

SECTION 1
NECK & JAW

These techniques release side of neck into shoulder and upper trapezius muscle.

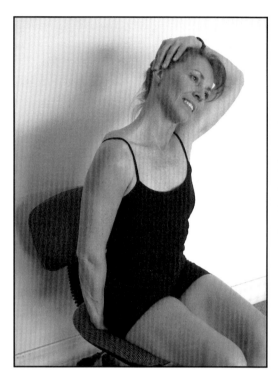

Anchor shoulder down by sitting on hand. Side-bend head to opposite direction. Try placing opposite hand on top of head and allowing it's weight to increase stretch on side of neck. Tilt chin slightly up or down to access different lines of restriction. **1-1**

Lengthen neck by lifting up through crown of head. Use shoulder muscles to actively depress shoulder.

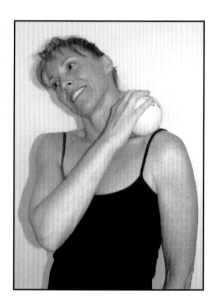

Shoulder can also be anchored down by pressing with opposite hand (not shown), or by pressing a ball into it. **1-2**

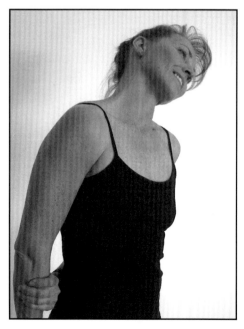

In standing, hold forearm with opposite hand and pull down to depress shoulder and elongate neck. **1-3**

These techniques release restrictions on back/side of neck into shoulder, including levator scapulae muscle.

As you release your neck, notice if your attention is drawn to any place else in your body. If so, work there next. If not, keep working your neck from all sides.

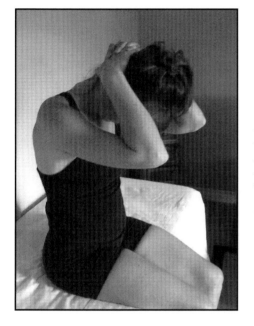

Sit tall. Clasp hands behind base of head. Allow gravity and weight of arms to elongate tissue, while actively lengthening back of neck. Experiment with slight rotation to either direction. Try in slumped position to allow stretch to expand into upper and possibly lower back. **1-4**

Sit on left hand to anchor shoulder down. Turn head 45 degrees right. Tuck chin to chest. With right palm on top of head, align forearm with nose and allow weight of right hand and active lengthening of neck through crown of head to increase stretch. From this position, try tilting chin slightly right or left to access different lines of restriction. Actively depress shoulder to further elongate tissue. **1-5**

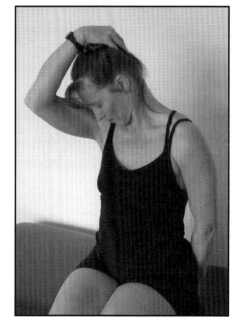

www.MyofascialStretching.com

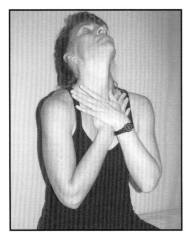

These techniques release restrictions in front of neck and throat, or scalene and hyoid muscles. They may help relieve TMJ dysfunction, jaw tightness, and teeth clenching and grinding.

Place one palm over other under clavicles. Sink in to anchor tissue. Tilt head back without allowing hands to slide. Allow gravity and weight of arms to maintain downward pressure while feeling stretch through front of neck. Try with mouth open and closed. **1-6**

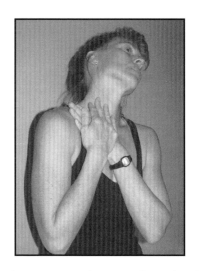

Place one palm over other under clavicles off to one side. Sink in to anchor tissue. Extend head back and side-bend in opposite direction. Try tilting chin up or down slightly to access different lines of restriction in fascial system. Also try with mouth open and closed. **1-7**

Can use ball to anchor tissue instead of hands. **1-8**

Compress palms into tissue on side of face. Palmer side of knuckles should sink into hollow between jaw and cheekbones. Allow weight of arms and gravity to decompress jaw, without allowing hands to slide down face. **1-9**

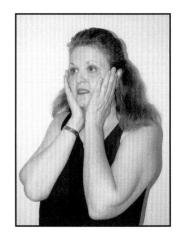

SECTION 2
SHOULDER

These techniques release tight shoulder blade muscles, especially rhomboids, middle trapezius, and levator scapulae.

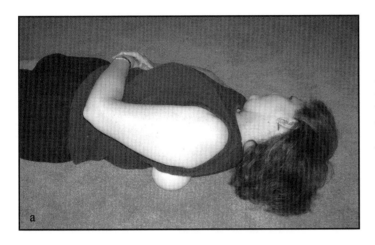

Lie on back with ball toward inside of shoulder blade. Find areas of tightness, pain or tension (a).

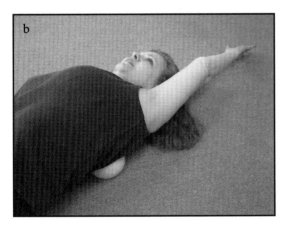
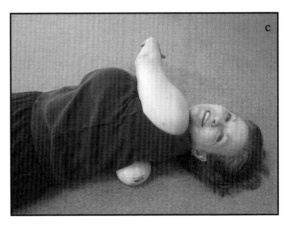

Elongate arm overhead (b) or across body (c) to increase stretch. **2-1**

*Place ball under area of pain or tightness.
Slowly roll on it to find point of greatest intensity.
Go slowly or you may pass right over a key spot.
When you find an area that is hot, hard or tender,
stay there and allow your body to sink further into ball.*

These techniques release restrictions in back of shoulder or posterior deltoid.

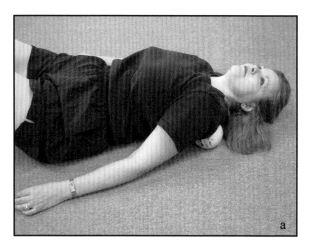 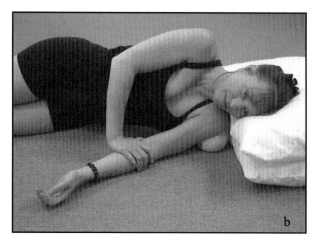

Lie on back (a) or side (b), with ball under back of shoulder. Relax into area of tightness. May use pillow under head to increase comfort. **2-2**

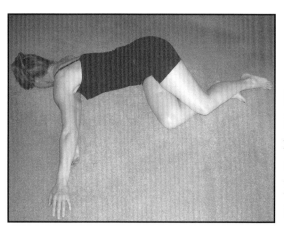

Lie on right side with right arm straight in front at 90 degrees. Left arm is on top of right arm. Slowly roll onto stomach, allowing left arm to slide along right arm. Lift head off surface to increase stretch on shoulder. **2-3**

Breathe. Relax. Melt.

Bring arm across body. Grasp back of shoulder with opposite hand (try holding over or under) and assist arm pull across body, further elongating tissue on back of shoulder. May also feel this in upper back. **2-4**

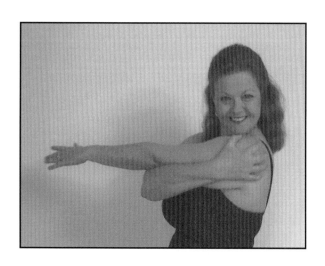

These techniques release pectoralis region in front of chest, ribcage, shoulder and armpit.

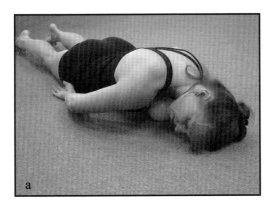
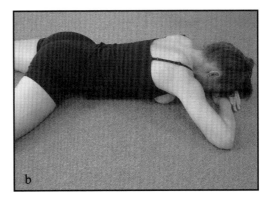

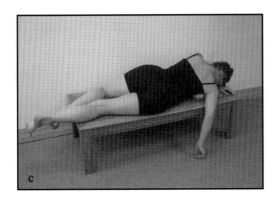

Lie on stomach with ball under front of ribs on anterior chest. Find areas of tightness or tenderness and relax into them. Try with arm down (a), overhead (b) or dropped off side of table or bed (c). **2-5**

Stay fully present with what you are feeling.

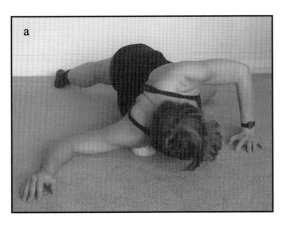
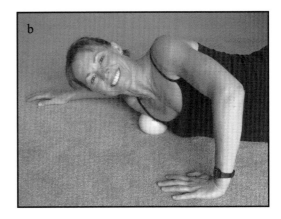

Lie on stomach with ball under ribs just inside front of shoulder. With shoulder and elbow both bent to 90 degrees and elbow out to side at shoulder height, roll rest of body away from floor (top shoulder towards ceiling). Drop top leg behind to elongate into stretch. (a) and (b) show the same stretch from two angles. **2-6**

www.MyofascialStretching.com

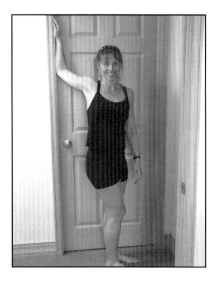

> *These techniques release pectoralis region in front of chest, ribcage, shoulder and armpit*

With right shoulder and elbow each bent to about 90 degrees and braced against door jam, rotate body in opposite direction and hold. Consider grasping opposite door jam with other hand for support or to help increase elongation (not shown). **2-7**

> *Find the pain. Look elsewhere for the cause.*

With arm overhead at a comfortable level, elbow straight and palm against door jam, rotate body in opposite direction and hold. Continue to turn body further away from arm as tissue releases (a).

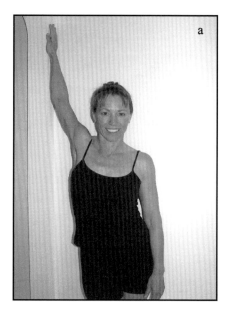

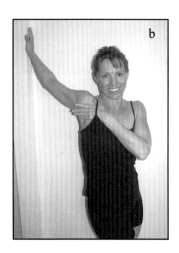
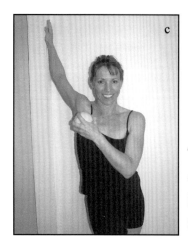

Try using opposite hand (b) or ball (c) to anchor tissue in front of ribcage, shoulder and armpit. **2-8**

18 www.MyofascialStretching.com

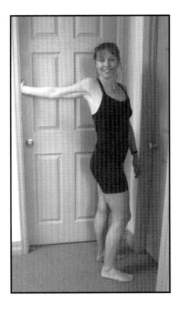

These techniques release restrictions in arm and front of shoulder, including biceps tendon.

With palm against door jam, rotate body in opposite direction and hold. Don't allow shoulder to rotate forward. Telescope arm and make it longer. Feel stretch in forearm, arm and front of shoulder. **2-9**

Stay with a technique as long as it continues to feel helpful. Wait patiently at the fascial barrier until you feel the release. Elongate further and wait again.

Clasp hands behind back. Kneel with clasped hands resting on table or back of couch. Lift chest and arch back to elongate into stretch. **2-10**

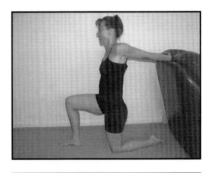

Can also do on back of chair while sitting in it at desk. **2-11**

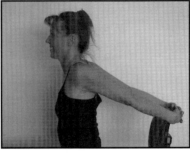

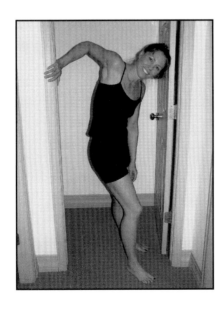

Place palm on doorway about shoulder height, fingers facing down and elbow higher than hand and shoulder. Bend down and lean forward into stretch, while rotating body slightly in opposite direction. Feel this directly in anterior shoulder and biceps tendon. **2-12**

www.MyofascialStretching.com

These techniques release chest, scapula, ribcage and front of shoulders.

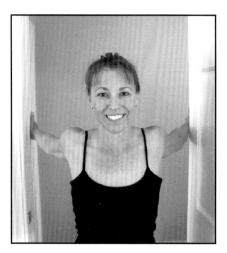

With both hands grasping opposing door jams, lean forward and hold. Lift chest and squeeze shoulder blades together to elongate further. **2-13**

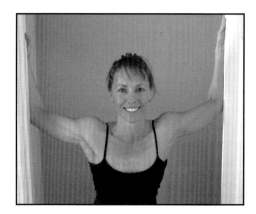

With both elbows bent to 90 degrees and at shoulder height, place palms against door jam. Lean forward, lift chest and squeeze shoulder blades together to elongate further into stretch. **2-14**

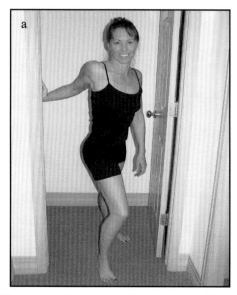

Place palm on doorway about shoulder height, elbow behind and slightly below level of shoulder (a). Lean forward into stretch and rotate body slightly in opposite direction. Feel this in front of shoulder, side of ribcage, and/or middle of back next to shoulder blade.

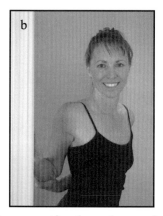

Try actively lowering elbow or pulling it down to further elongate or access different areas of restriction (b). **2-15**

*These techniques release
back of armpit and lateral border of shoulder blade,
including subscapularis and latissimus dorsi.*

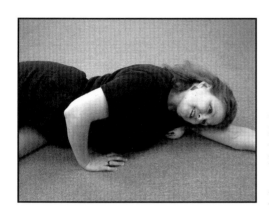

*Remember to hold every stretch
a minimum of 90 to 120 seconds,
or until you feel a release.*

Lie on side with ball towards back of armpit. Find area of tightness or tenderness and relax and soften into it. Reach or elongate arm to increase stretch where ball is pressing. **2-16**

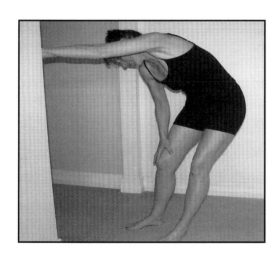

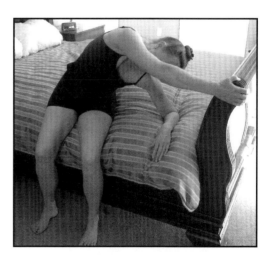

Bend forward and grasp door jam with one hand. Lean back and elongate to feel stretch in back of armpit and shoulder blade. Try subtle weight shifts and leaning in different directions to access different lines of restriction. Experiment with palm facing in or out. **2-17**

Sit on edge of bed resting on one elbow. Reach across body to grasp footboard with hand. Lean away. Elongate trunk and arm to feel stretch in back of armpit and shoulder blade. Repeat with other side. Great stretch to do when getting out of bed in morning. **2-18**

SECTION 3
UPPER EXTREMITY

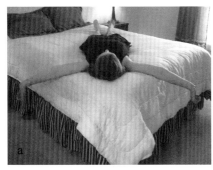

These techniques release restrictions throughout entire arm, especially biceps, forearm, wrist and hand.

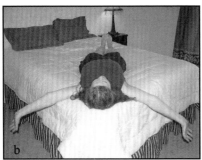

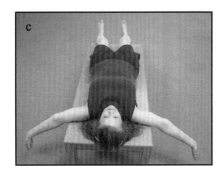

Lie diagonally on corner of bed, or on coffee table with arms supported up to elbows. While keeping arms resting on bed or table, actively telescope or lengthen them. Extend wrists backwards and engage fascial barrier at tolerable intensity. Hold at least several minutes. Continue to extend wrists further as tissue releases. Experiment with fingers flexed, which will focus tension in forearm (a), or extended, which will focus tension in palmer surface of hand (b, c). **3-1**

After holding technique through several releases, roll arms inward, flex wrists and cone fingers to release back side of forearm and wrist (see 3-8 for example of position). **3-2**

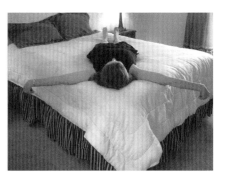

Reach. Telescope. Elongate.
Feel the tissue engaged along entire length of arm.
The fascial barrier is the point at which you feel resistance to the stretch.

These techniques release restrictions in forearm, wrist and hands, and mobilize median nerve.

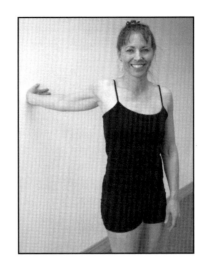

With palm placed flat against wall, extend arm and rotate body away from hand. Elongate through entire arm. **3-3**

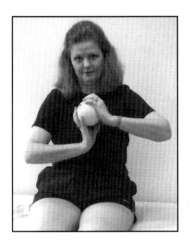

Place ball between hands and use pressure of one hand on ball to bend other hand backwards for wrist and forearm stretch. Roll ball onto tips of fingers to focus tension in hand. **3-4**

Sit tall with both hands draped over balls, behind line of body. Lift chest and arch back to elongate. Place balls further back to increase intensity of stretch. This elongates front of shoulders, biceps tendons, forearms, wrists and hands. **3-5**

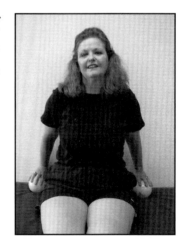

Follow the 'fascial voice'. Listen to your body. Where is it telling you to work next?

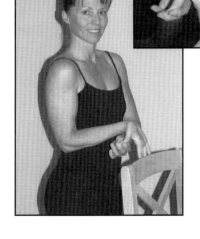

With elbow at 90 degrees and wrist bent back, push extended fingers into stable surface such as table or chair. Use opposite hand to put slight tension on thumb, releasing thenar fascia and mobilizing median nerve. **3-6**

www.MyofascialStretching.com

These techniques mobilize median, radial and ulnar nerves, in addition to releasing fascial restrictions in forearm, wrist and hand.

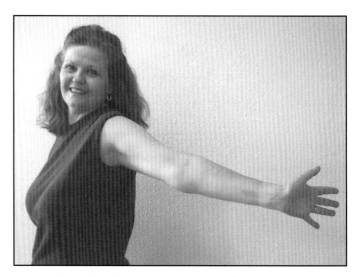

Can be done with one arm or both simultaneously.

Median Nerve: Stretch and elongate arm out to side. Actively extend wrist and fingers back. Feel tension along length of arm, forearm, wrist and hand. **3-7**

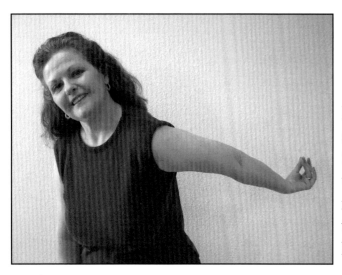

Try each technique in standing, sitting or lying down. The angle of tension may change slightly in different positions.

Radial Nerve: Stretch and telescope arm out to side. Bring shoulder forward, rotate arm internally, flex wrist and cone fingers, while maintaining elongation of arm. Feel tension along back of forearm and hand. **3-8**

Actively elongate head and neck away from arm being stretched.

Ulnar Nerve: Bend elbow with wrist bent backwards and fingers extended. Stretch and elongate through elbow, as if telescoping it away from body. Feel tension along front of forearm into little fingers. **3-9**

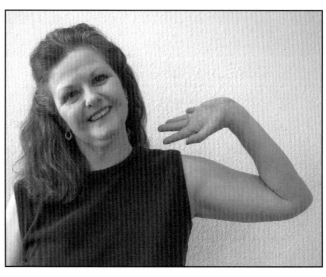

These techniques release restrictions under arm, or in tricep area.

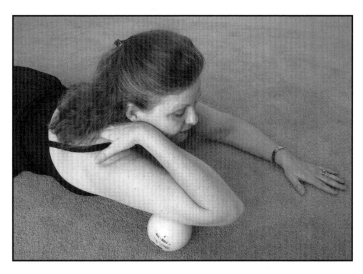

Lie on stomach with elbow bent and ball in fleshy area under arm in location of tightness or restriction. Elongate tissue by telescoping tip of elbow away from body. **3-10**

Maintain conscious awareness of what you are feeling. Direct your breath into the restriction.

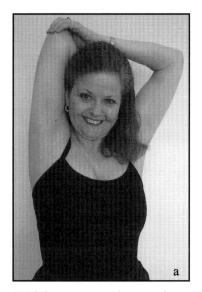

With arm elongating towards the ceiling and elbow bent, grasp tip of elbow with other hand and gently pull backwards to release back of arm (a).

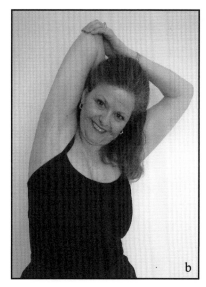

Elongate lateral trunk and focus of tension will move to armpit or side of trunk (b). **3-11**

www.MyofascialStretching.com

SECTION 4
LATERAL TRUNK

These techniques release restrictions in lateral trunk, rib cage and armpit/scapular area.

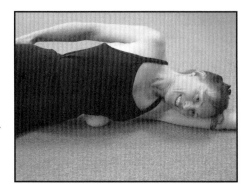

Lie on side with ball under tight or tender area of ribcage. Telescope arm and/or leg to increase stretch. **4-1**

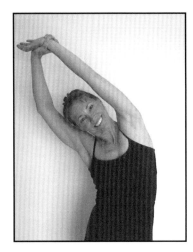

Grasp wrist with opposite hand. Pull overhead and across body, while actively elongating trunk. Try in sitting and standing. Sitting stretch will focus more in armpit and upper trunk. Standing stretch will focus tension lower in trunk and possibly into pelvis and hip. **4-2**

Reach. Elongate. Telescope.

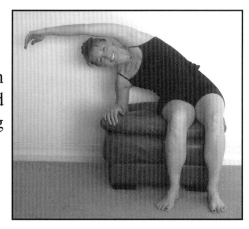

Sit on bench, bed, or ottoman, leaning on elbow. Reach overhead and elongate arm and lateral trunk to side. If on bed, try holding headboard or footboard to increase stretch. **4-3**

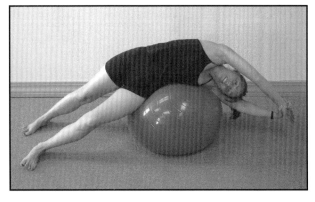

Lie sideways on large therapy ball. Allow body to drape over it. Elongate by telescoping top arm and leg. If balance is a concern, have someone spot you or do with ball in front of couch for support. **4-4**

SECTION 5
SPINE

These techniques release tightness and mobilize each segment of spinal column.

Spend the most time in areas that feel significant. Listen to your body.

Variation: Use two balls simultaneously on either side of spine to release soft tissue.

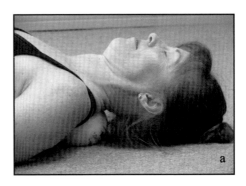
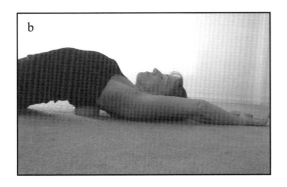
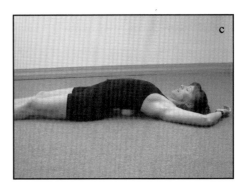
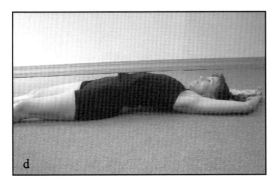
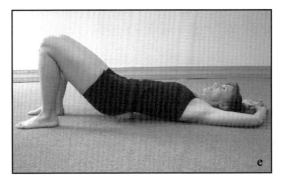

Lie with ball directly under spine (a). Start at top and move ball down spine ½ inch at a time. Try with arms down or elongated overhead with ball under upper back (b). Breathe and relax into each site until release occurs. This should eventually be done for all segments of spinal column, as it helps to mobilize spine (c). It is equally effective to start at base of spine and work upwards (d). Experiment with knees straight or bent with ball under lower back (e). **5-1**

www.MyofascialStretching.com

SECTION 6
UPPER & MID BACK

These techniques release upper and mid back, scapula, thorax, chest and ribcage.

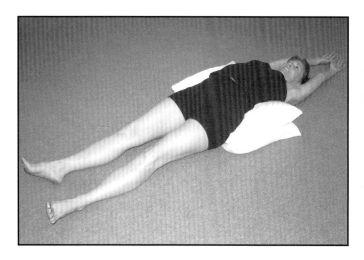

Lie on back with one or two thick pillows beneath mid back. Elongate arms overhead and telescope legs in opposite direction. Feel stretch in back, ribcage, anterior chest. **6-1**

A release may feel like taffy lengthening or butter melting. There may be a burning or ripping sensation, pulsing, tingling or a release of heat.

Sit tall on solid chair with a back, facing sideways. Grasp sides of chair back with hands and rotate body towards chair back. Elongate through upper body by sitting taller and maintain rotational tension through push/pulling of hands on chair back. Feel stretch in thorax, ribcage, front of shoulder or scapula, depending on your particular patterns of tightness. **6-2**

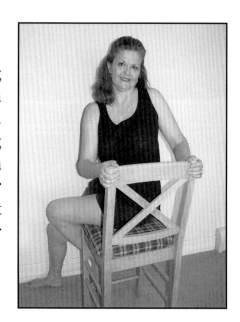

These techniques release upper/ mid back and scapula.

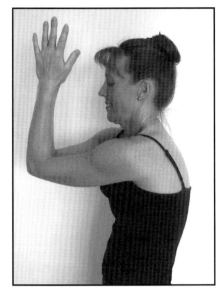

Place hands in prayer position with elbows bent to 90 degrees and close together at shoulder height. Actively round upper back and slide shoulder blades laterally around rib cage to elongate further. Feel stretch in upper back. **6-3**

Breathe into the restriction. Wait patiently at the barrier for tissue to release.

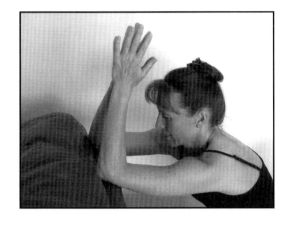

Try above technique sitting on chair with elbows on table. Slide chair back and lean forward, using table to lift elbows further to increase stretch. A great technique to do sitting at your desk. **6-4**

Remember to hold all stretches at least 90 to 120 seconds.

Cross arms and reach around back. Clasp hands behind shoulder blades. Round and elongate upper back while reaching even further around in a hug. **6-5**

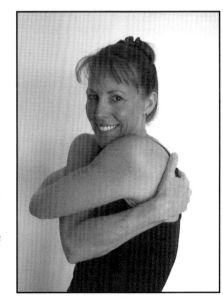

www.MyofascialStretching.com

SECTION 7
LOW BACK

These techniques release restrictions in low back, abdominal obliques and quadratus areas.

Breathe, relax and sink into ball. Imagine cheese melting over a hamburger as your tissue softens.

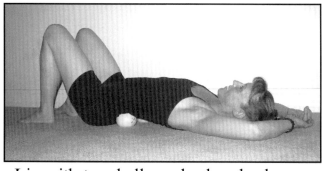

Lie with two balls under low back, on either side of spine. Bend knees to increase ball pressure in low back. **7-1**

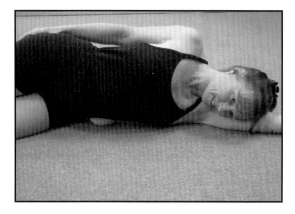

Lie on side with ball under area of tightness or tenderness. Allow arm to act as pillow for head. Elongate arm and/or leg. Roll slightly forward or back to seek out restriction. **7-2**

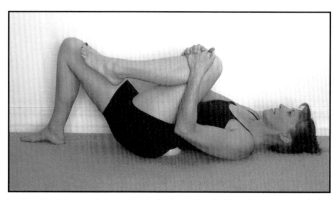

Lie on back with ball just above pelvis, 3-4 inches to side of spine under tight or tender area. Flex hip and knee on same side, pulling knee towards chest. Actively elongate lower back. **7-3**

> *These techniques release restrictions in low back, abdominal obliques and quadratus areas.*

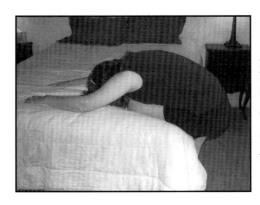

Flex knees and hips with feet and buttocks hanging off edge of bed and arms stretched overhead. Round and elongate through entire back. **7-4**

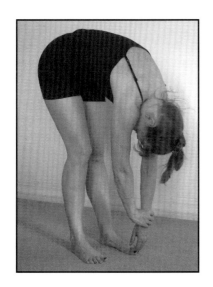

Keep left leg straight and bend right leg slightly. Flex forward at hips, rotating away from straight leg. Grasp left wrist and pull towards floor and to right, while actively elongating through low back. Feel stretch on left low back. **7-5**

> *It is not uncommon to spend 3 to 5 minutes on one technique.*

With right leg straight and left foot up on chair, bend forward at hips. Grasp left wrist and pull or elongate towards floor. Feel stretch in left low back or buttock. May also feel in inner thigh. **7-6**

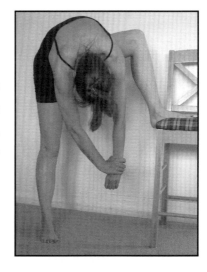

www.MyofascialStretching.com 31

SECTION 8
ABDOMEN & FRONT OF HIP

These techniques release restrictions in abdominal and pelvic floor areas, including psoas and oblique musculature, and can be helpful for low back pain.

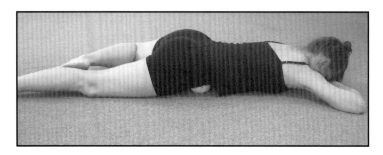

Lie face down with ball just to inside of pelvic bone under area of tightness. Leg on opposite side is rotated outwards with knee bent. Explore entire pelvic floor area for restrictions. **8-1**

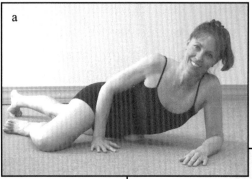

Lie on side with upper body resting on elbow with ball just above and inside of pelvic bone, on area of tightness (a). Elongate through lower trunk.

Be present with what you are feeling.

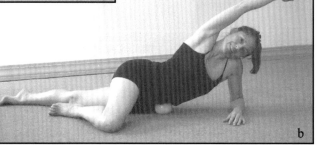

Experiment with other arm position.
Reach overhead, for example (b). **8-2**

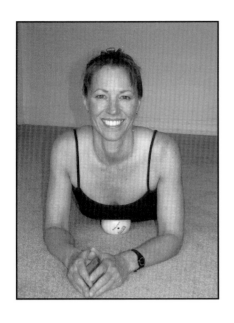

These techniques release restrictions in abdominal and pelvic floor areas, including psoas and oblique musculature, and can be helpful for low back pain.

Lie on stomach with ball directly under midline. Start just under ribs and move ball down about one inch at a time, softening in each area. It may be necessary to come up on elbows to lessen intensity, or to start out on a softer surface. **8-3**

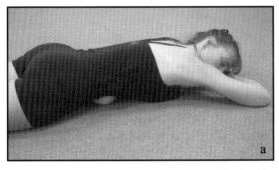

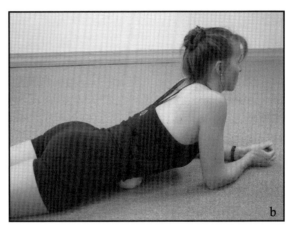

Lie on stomach and start with ball one inch above and to side of navel. Breathe, relax and allow tissue to soften over ball. Move ball down abdomen about one inch at a time, into pelvic bowl, staying about one inch to side of midline or navel (a).

Try propped on elbows to elongate abdominal fascia (b). **8-4**

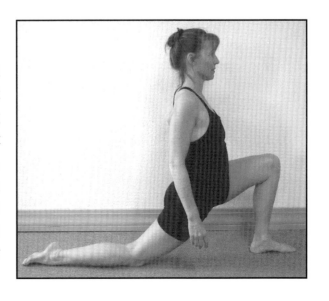

Bend left hip and knee in front and extend right leg behind. Tighten right buttock and elongate or lengthen right leg further. Feel stretch in front of right abdomen, hip or thigh. As fascia releases, get taller through trunk and elongate leg further. Works well using ski poles (see Jill's preface) or furniture on both sides to support upper body and allow further sinking into stretch. **8-5**

www.MyofascialStretching.com

These techniques release restrictions in front of hip and quadriceps and can be helpful for low back pain.

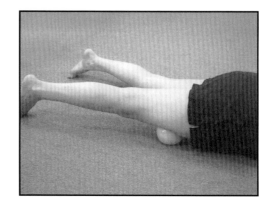

Lie on stomach with ball under front of thigh in area of tightness, allowing tissue to melt over ball. Elongate leg to enhance stretch. **8-6**

Quality is more important than quantity. It is of greater benefit to go deeply into one technique than to race through several quickly.

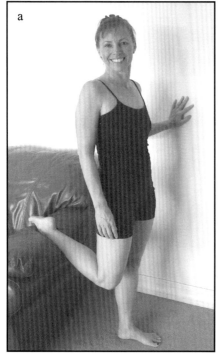

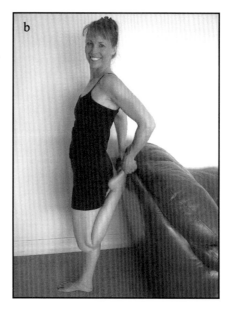

Stand tall in front of piece of furniture. Bend knee and rest top of foot on furniture for support. Keep knees together, and elongate bent knee towards floor. Actively lift hip on side being stretched to level it with other one. Feel stretch in front of thigh. Choose furniture height based on flexibility (a, b). **8-7**

Look for props in your environment to facilitate Myofascial Stretching.

These techniques release restrictions in front of hip and quadriceps and can be helpful for low back pain.

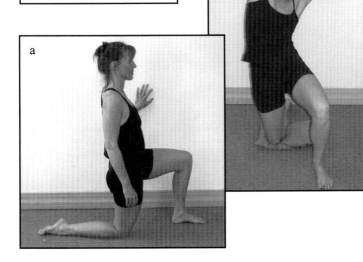

Active elongation through hip joint is key to these stretches.

In half kneeling position, stabilize self with hand on wall or furniture. Tighten right buttock and lengthen tissue in front of hip and thigh by kneeling as tall as possible. Try to push right hip forward without actually leaning forward by tightening right buttock even further and pulling grounded left foot toward you without actually moving foot (a). Reach overhead with right arm to increase stretch along front of hip and lateral trunk. Use left arm to assist. Can use pillow under knee for comfort (b). **8-8**

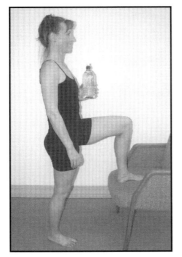

Stand tall with left foot on chair, elongating tissue throughout length of standing right leg. Tighten right buttock muscles and pull left foot towards you without actually moving it, creating an elongation stretch in front of right hip. **8-9**

Keep your attention focused on maintaining tension at the fascial barrier.

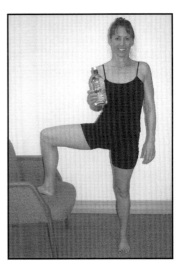

Stand tall with right foot to side on chair, elongating tissue throughout length of standing left leg. Tighten left buttock muscles and pull right foot towards you without actually moving it, creating an elongation stretch along inner left thigh. **8-10**

www.MyofascialStretching.com

SECTION 9
HIPS & BUTTOCKS

These techniques release restrictions in buttocks, including piriformis and gluteal musculature.

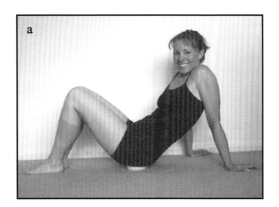 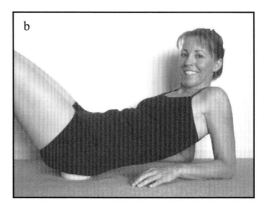

Sit propped on arms with ball under tight area of buttock (a). After finding and releasing several restrictions, lower upper body onto elbow and find new areas of tension (b). Explore all the way up to pelvic crest. **9-1**

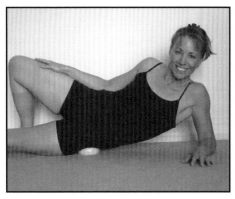

Roll more to side to find any restrictions in lateral buttock or hip. **9-2**

Modify the intensity by lying on a harder or softer surface.

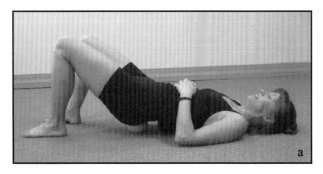 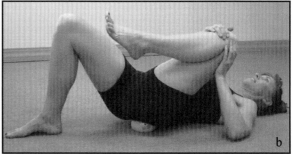

Finally, lie flat on back with ball under buttock and allow body to soften over ball (a). Try flexing hip and pulling knee towards you to further elongate into stretch (b). **9-3**

These techniques release restrictions in buttocks, including piriformis and gluteal musculature.

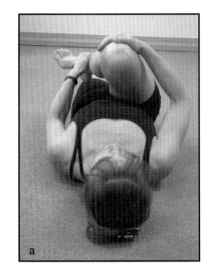

Lie on back with left leg extended and right knee and hip flexed. Hold right knee at midline of body with right hand. Hold right ankle with left hand and gently pull ankle toward you, rotating hip. Feel stretch in right buttock. As tissue releases, pull knee further towards midline or past it and pull ankle in closer. (a) and (b) are different angles of same stretch. **9-4**

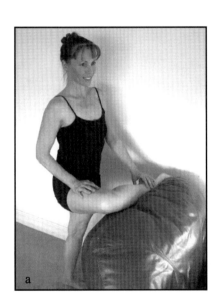

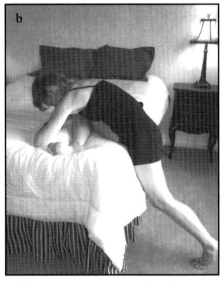

Stand tall, lengthening muscles of left leg, with right leg resting on bed or back of couch, with knee bent and hip externally rotated (a). Feel stretch in right buttock. Stand taller to elongate further into stretch as tissue releases. Bend forward to change stretch and line of tension.

Eventually, rest upper body on leg if flexibility allows (b). Try changing position of right leg, moving it further to right or left of upper body to access different lines of restriction. **9-5**

These techniques release restrictions in inner, back, and outer thighs including adductors, hamstrings, and IT bands.

SECTION 10
UPPER LEG

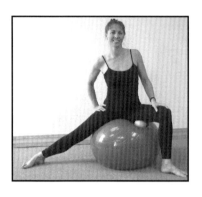
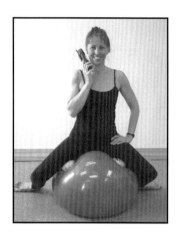
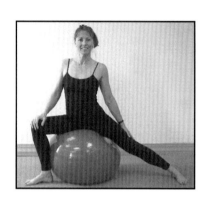

Sit on large therapy ball with small ball under tight inner thigh. Experiment with varying positions in order to elongate tissue further. For example, lean or shift weight forward using furniture for support, bend or straighten and telescope leg, rotate body, try two balls at once. Eventually shift ball lower towards knee, then more under central thigh, and finally under outer thigh. **10-1**

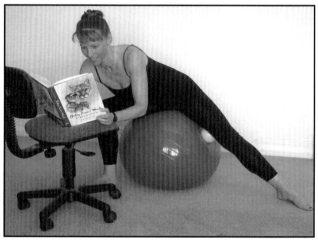

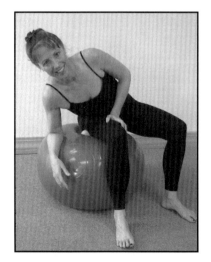

You may find it more comfortable wearing long pants while doing these techniques.

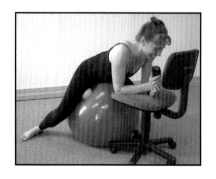
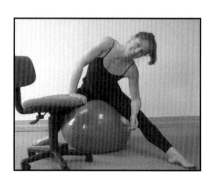

38 www.MyofascialStretching.com

These techniques release restrictions in inner thighs including adductors and inner hamstrings.

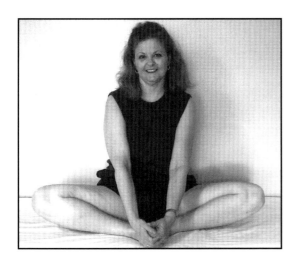

Sitting tall, place bottoms of feet together and gently pull them towards you. Feel stretch on inner thighs. Continue to elongate by sitting taller and pulling feet further towards you to access additional layers of restriction. **10-2**

Spread legs with back foot pointing forward and front leg externally rotated with front foot pointing to side, or perpendicular to back foot. Shift weight sideways towards front leg and feel stretch along inner thigh of front leg. Bend forward to further elongate and rest upper body on piece of furniture. Telescope and lengthen through front leg. **10-3**

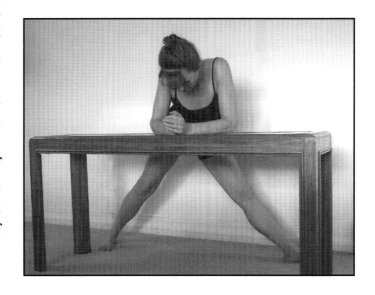

Breathe deeply, imagining the breath flowing to areas of pain and restriction. Relax. Let go and soften your body. Never force the tissue. Maintain the stretch at the barrier and wait for a release to occur.

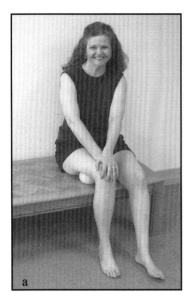

These techniques release restrictions in back of thighs, hamstrings and into calves.

Sit on bench or table with ball under tight area of thigh. Shift weight forward or back, side to side to find area of tension. Stay there, relaxing and allowing tissue to melt over ball. Explore entire back of thigh (a). Find restriction with ball under lateral thigh and lean sideways, resting on elbow to elongate and increase intensity (b). Reach arm overhead to further increase stretch (c). **10-4**

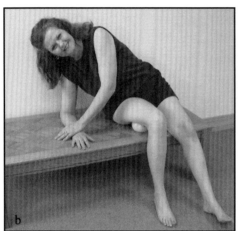
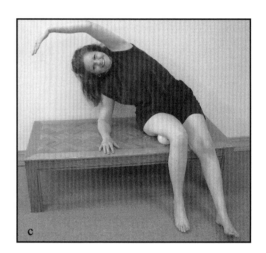

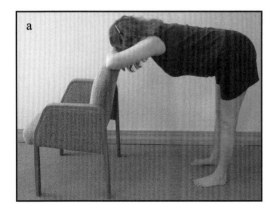
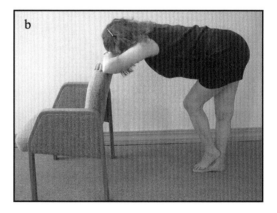

Lean forward and rest upper body on chair or table. Lift tailbone toward ceiling and drop lower back towards floor. Feel stretch in back of legs. As tissue releases, allow body to shift forward, back or to side to access next layer of restriction. Actively lower back further towards floor, while lifting tailbone higher to increase elongation. Try both legs together (a), or one leg at a time with non-weight bearing foot resting on top of weight bearing foot (b). **10-5**

These techniques release restrictions in lateral thigh, including IT band.

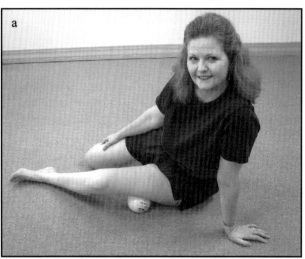

Side-sit with ball in area of restriction under outside of thigh. Keep weight over ball (a).

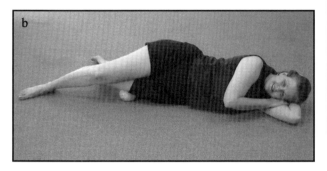

To increase intensity, lie on side with lower leg straight and elongated and upper leg in front of lower leg to bring weight over ball (b).

Use ball to release entire area from hip down to knee.

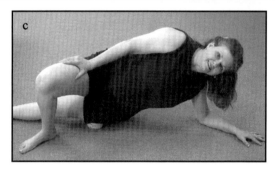

Come up on elbow to increase intensity even further (c). **10-6**

Keep the intensity mild to moderate in order to stay with the technique long enough for the tissue to release.

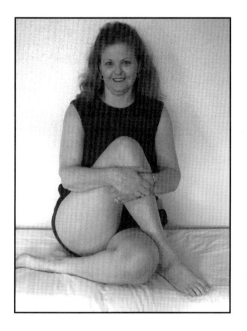

Sit tall with left knee flexed so foot is nearly under right hip. Cross right leg over left with knee up and right foot next to left knee. Clasp hands or arms around right knee and gently pull towards chest. Feel stretch in right thigh, hip or buttock. As tissue releases, pull knee closer to body and sit even taller to access next layer of restriction. **10-7**

SECTION 11
LOWER LEG

These techniques release restrictions in tops of feet and shins, including tibialis anterior.

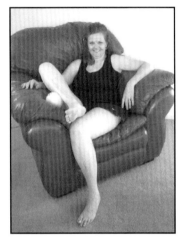

*Remember:
Always work on both sides of body, even if symptoms are only on one.*

Sit in relaxed position in easy chair with tight area of lateral front of shin resting on ball. **11-1**

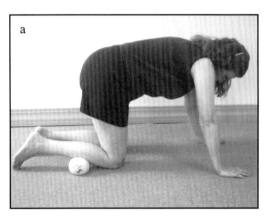
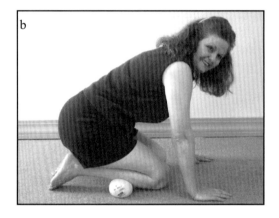

Kneel on all fours with tight area of lateral front of shin resting on ball (a). Sit back on heels to increase intensity (b). **11-2**

While sitting in chair, tuck toes under and rest them on floor to release tops of feet and shins. Can be done while working at desk or on computer. **11-3**

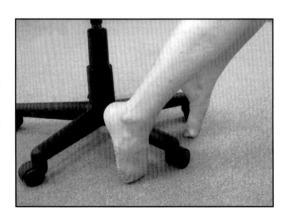

These techniques release restrictions in calves.

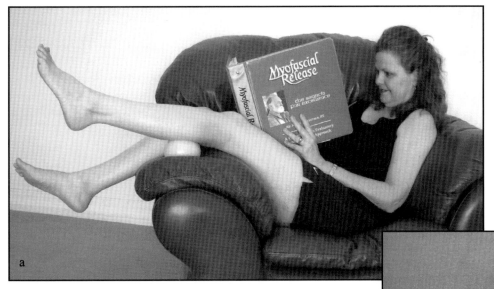

Place ball under tight part of calf. Can be accomplished in various positions as shown (a, b). **11-4**

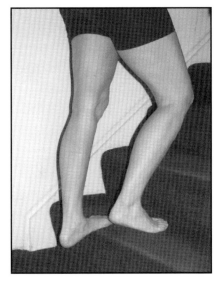

Stand with most of weight on ball of one foot on edge of stair with heel hanging off. Hold on to rail for support. Actively lower heel further to increase stretch. Try with knee straight and knee bent. May work better with shoes on if balls of feet are sensitive. **11-5**

Squat on one leg, with other bent leg resting out to side. Rest hands or forearms on knee and center weight of upper body over knee to increase stretch through lower calf. Actively lower heel towards floor. **11-6**

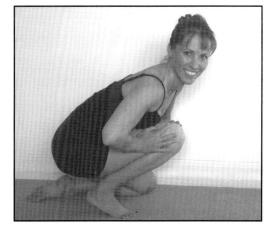

This technique releases restrictions in fascial sheath along back of legs, particularly in calves.

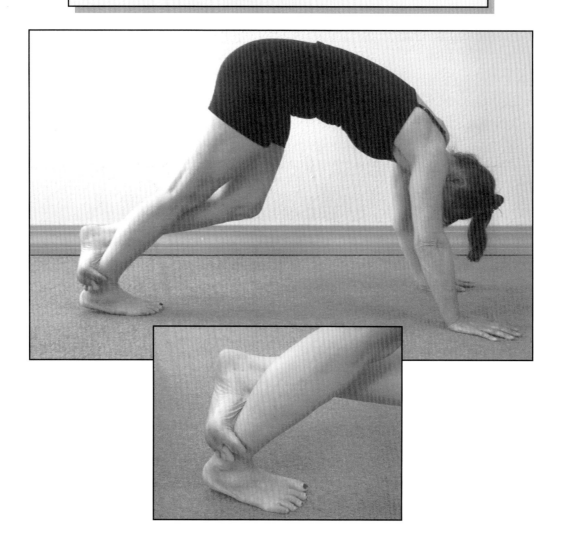

With hips flexed and hands and both feet on floor, feel stretch in back of legs and calves (not shown). Rest one foot on other ankle to focus on one calf at a time. Actively elongate by lifting opposite hip so it is level with weight bearing one. Lengthen calf further by lowering heel towards floor. Hold at least 90 to 120 seconds. **11-7**

*Enter into and exit out of all stretches slowly and consciously.
When you find the fascial restriction
engage it at the barrier by elongating further.
Follow the tissue as it releases into the next barrier.
Remember, there are always multiple layers of restriction.*

This series of techniques releases restrictions in lateral and top portions of feet, calves, shins, and back of thighs.

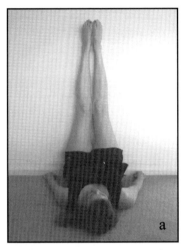

Point toes towards ceiling and feel stretch in tops of feet and front of shins (a).

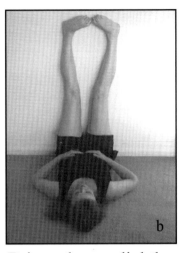

Bring legs slightly apart and roll feet in to lengthen lateral aspect of feet and calves (b).

Lie with hips as close to wall as possible and legs telescoping towards ceiling.

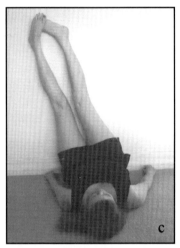

Slide legs off to one side and use one foot to press on toes of other foot to elongate tissue on lateral aspect of foot and calf (c).

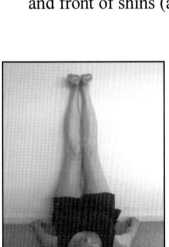

Bring legs back to center and pull toes towards you (d).

Hold each position at least 90 to 120 seconds.

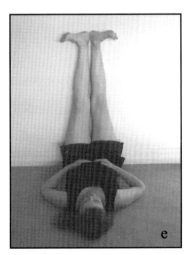

With toes pulled towards you, rotate feet outwards to change line of stretch (e).

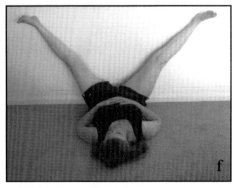

Slide legs out along wall and release inner thighs (f). **11-8**

www.MyofascialStretching.com   45

*These techniques
release restrictions
in bottoms of feet and toes.*

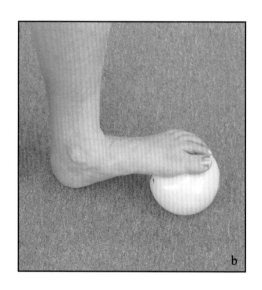

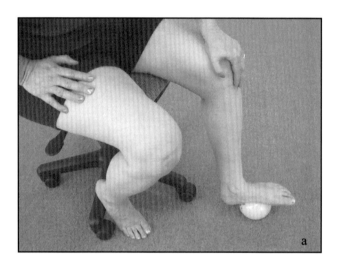

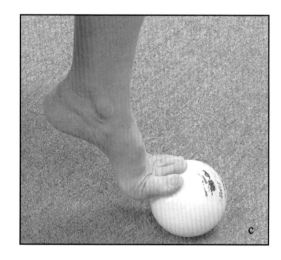

Sit with arch of foot resting on ball (a). Relax and allow foot to soften around ball. After tissue releases, move ball under ball of foot and relax and soften again (b). Finally, move ball under bent toes to stretch toes and ball of foot (c). These can be done while sitting at a desk or working on a computer. The last one can also be done anywhere without the ball (d). Hold each position at least 90 to 120 seconds. **11-9**

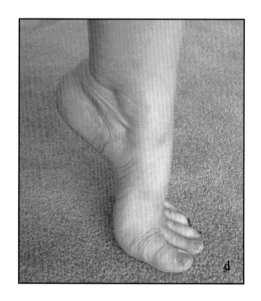

*Make Myofascial Stretching
a part of your daily life,
whenever and wherever you can.
Focus your awareness
on what your body is feeling
as you go about your activities.*

SECTION 12
MULTIPLE RELEASE TECHNIQUES

If balance is a concern, have someone spot you or do with ball in between couch and coffee table for support.

The following techniques release restrictions in so many areas, they deserve their own category. These ball stretches are great to do after any forward bending activity which is likely to result in back discomfort such as vacuuming, shoveling, mowing the lawn, or typing at the computer.

To get on and off ball: Start by sitting on therapy ball.
Walk feet out until lying on ball in desired location (upper/mid/low back).
When finished, walk feet back towards ball until once again sitting on it.
Sit for a moment before standing up to avoid light-headedness or dizziness.

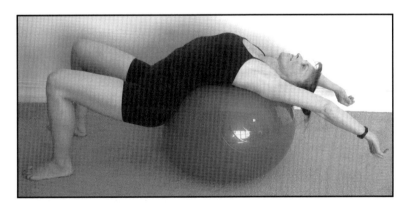

Lie with therapy ball under upper back. Elongate arms to side or overhead, depending on flexibility and desired area of stretch. Allow body to soften and drape over ball. Breathe and relax into stretch in upper and mid back, anterior chest, ribcage and shoulders. When ready, walk feet back in until sitting on ball again. **12-1**

www.MyofascialStretching.com

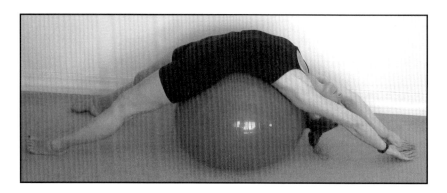

Redo last stretch with therapy ball under mid back. Continue to elongate arms overhead. Straighten legs and telescope towards feet. Feel stretch again in upper and mid back, anterior chest, ribcage and shoulders. In addition, low back, abdomen and front of hips should feel some lengthening. **12-2**

> If neck feels stressed,
> place small pillow or rolled up towel under it.

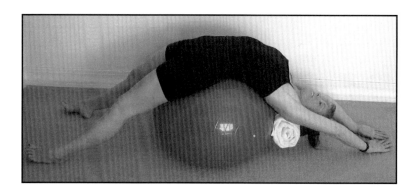

Move therapy ball under low back. Continue to elongate arms overhead, and telescope straight legs towards feet. Feel this stretch in mid and low back, chest and ribcage, abdomen, front of hips and inner thighs. **12-3**

> Start by doing these techniques separately.
> Over time, as body softens, releases and gets used to inverted position,
> do all three positions in one sequence.

*This technique releases restrictions in arm, armpit and shoulder blade.
Or, with a slightly different focus,
it releases tightness off to side of spine in low back,
including quadratus lumborum.*

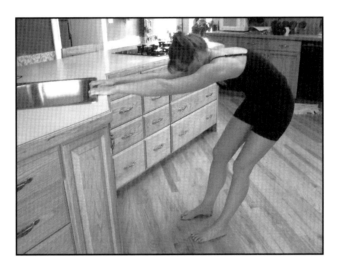

The Kitchen Sink Release

Bend forward, grasping edge of sink with fingers of both hands. Lean back and feel for areas of tightness. Adjust body weight and position to focus stretch in arms and shoulders, one or both sides at a time. Elongate through upper back and arms until release occurs.

Now, adjust position to concentrate stretch to one side of low back. Place most of body weight through left arm and leg. Elongate through left middle and low back, focusing on lengthening tissue on left side of back. Tuck pelvis and tailbone under to further increase stretch. **12-4**

*Use your imagination to find props at home, at the office
or provided by Mother Nature. This book is just a starting point.
Develop your own techniques. There are no right or wrong positions.
Just follow the basic principles and you will be able to
release fascial restrictions throughout your body.*

ABOUT THE AUTHORS

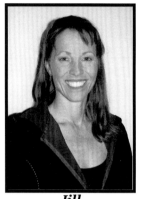
Jill

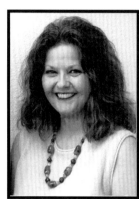
Brenda

Jill Stedronsky, MS, OTR

With nearly twenty years of experience as an Occupational Therapist, Jill has worked in a variety of rehabilitation settings. Her training includes all Myofascial Release courses taught by John F. Barnes, PT; CranioSacral, Lymph Drainage, SomatoEmotional Release and Pediatrics courses from the Upledger Institute; Manual Therapy, Motor Control, Neural Mobilization, Cranial and Spinal Mobilization, Orthopedic and Muscle Energy Techniques from Manual Therapy Seminars; and Healing Touch courses from the Colorado Center for Healing Touch. She blends these approaches with soft tissue mobilization, neuromuscular re-education, movement and postural awareness, and home exercise programs. She believes in empowering her clients by teaching home exercises to enhance and maintain the benefits gained through therapy. Jill has found that combining hands-on therapy with self-treatment is a highly successful and cost effective method to reduce pain, restore function and enhance the well being of her clients. Jill has private practices in Denver and Lakewood, Colorado.

Brenda Pardy, OTR

In her more than thirty years as an Occupational Therapist, Brenda has experience treating adults and children with neurologic, orthopedic, and developmental issues. Since taking her first courses in John Barnes' method of Myofascial Release, she has changed the focus of her treatment to include these techniques along with more traditional modalities and Sensory Integration Therapy. Brenda has found that the addition of this innovative whole-body approach has increased the rate of improvement and the longevity of the results for her patients. She has resolved her own neck and back pain with Myofascial Release Treatment and Myofascial Stretching. Brenda's repertoire of treatment approaches also includes CranioSacral Therapy, Visceral Manipulation, Quantum Touch and High Touch Jin Shin. She is the director of the Physical and Occupational Therapy Departments at both Greenwood Therapy Institute and Pediatric Therapy Institute.

What people are saying about

MYOFASCIAL STRETCHING
A Guide to Self-Treatment

Finally a resource that truly helps to empower patients. Myofascial Stretching is a wonderful therapeutic tool and a valuable reference for therapists and patients alike. This easy to use book clearly explains and demonstrates effective use of treatment balls for release of myofascial tissues and structural balance. The innovative way these concepts are incorporated into daily activities makes the approach easy and effective. The techniques are an integral component of a comprehensive manual physical therapy program.   **-Sandra Do, DPT, FAAOMPT, OCS,** *Owner/ Manual Therapy Associates, Inc.*

As an athlete who runs half-marathons, I was doing fine with only minimal aches and pains. After purchasing Myofascial Stretching with the 4" ball and using them at my office, I run faster and feel looser and more fluid. My overall outlook on life has improved from doing these simple yet effective techniques every day. How can I not feel great about myself when I feel so good? I am using the ball as I write. Thanks to Jill and Brenda along with John Barnes for getting this message out to all.
-John M. Murphy, *Information Technology Specialist*

I use Myofascial Stretching exercises myself, with my Pilates students, and all my personal training clients. Everyone progresses exponentially from this unique approach to stretching.
-Katie Thornhill, BS, C-PT, PTA, CPI, *Owner/Personal Pilates Plus, Inc.*

The Self-Treatment Stretching Guide is a wonderful tool to help patients maintain benefits of Myofascial Release between treatments. The pictures and detailed instructions provide the clarity needed for patients to follow through on home programs. Jill and Brenda did a great job and people are loving it.
-Lorie Legatski, OTR, *Owner/Therapeutic Relief, Inc.*

The step-by-step instructions and clear photographs are easy to follow. Instead of calling my doctor when I have a new ache or pain, I look in the book and can often resolve the issue on my own. I highly recommend this book to family, friends and colleagues.   **-Jo Klein,** *Fiber Artist, Educator*

Breast cancer and surgeries left my body weak, in pain and dysfunctional. Despite working out with a personal trainer, I became more constricted and less flexible. My doctor suggested Myofascial Release. Jill treated me and gave me stretches from this book. I now have full, pain free range of motion and my self-confidence back. Myofascial Stretching was an important part of my rehabilitation and still makes a wonderful difference in my life to this day.   **-Joan Gitchell, RN, MS, SNP,** *Retired School Nurse*

Myofascial Stretching is extraordinary! You can practice it anywhere: at home, office, or a serene beach. Experience transformation thru elongation of the very fibers that embrace your soul. Myofascial Stretching facilitates a deeper connection with body, mind and spirit. I recommend it for everyone. This is truly a gift.   **-Janet Nicole Sykora, MA, OTR,** *Owner/Medical Professional Connections, Inc.*
Certified Indoor Cycling Instructor, AAAI/ISMA

INFORMATION

For information on hosting a Myofascial Stretching Course,
or to experience Myofascial Release Treatment
in the Denver, Colorado area,
please contact one of the authors.

Jill Stedronsky, MS, OTR
303 332 9171
Jill@DenverMyofascialRelease.com

Brenda Pardy, OTR
Greenwood Therapy Institute
303 649 9007
Brenda@DenverMyofascialRelease.com

Visit their website at
www.DenverMyofascialRelease.com

To order Myofascial Stretching Books and Balls:

- Call 303 649 9007 ext #3
- Order directly online at www.MyofascialStretching.com
- Fill out order form in back of book and either mail or fax it
- Email your order to StretchingBook@MyofascialStretching.com
- Download an order form from www.MyofascialStretching.com and mail or fax it

Bulk discounts are available on books.

To learn more about Myofascial Release,
order John Barnes' books,
or find a therapist near you
visit the official website at
www.MyofascialRelease.com

MYOFASCIAL STRETCHING
A Guide to Self-Treatment

Order Form

Item	Price	Quantity	Amount
Myofascial Stretching Book			
1-9 $ 29.99 each			
10-24 $ 24.99 each			
25 or more $ 19.99 each			
4" Inflatable Ball (Standard) $ 5.00 each			
3" Inflatable Ball* $ 4.00 each			
5" Inflatable Ball* $ 6.00 each			
*See the Tool section on Page 7 for a description of when to use alternative sized balls.			

One of each size ball $12.99

	Subtotal	$

Make Checks Payable and Mail to:
Denver Myofascial Release
6535 South Dayton Street
Suite 3800
Greenwood Village, CO 80111

Shipping & Handling	
Please call or visit our website for shipping and handling information	
CO residents 7.35 % tax	$
Total	$

Phone Orders and Inquiries: 303-649-9007
Fax Form to: 303-649-9008

Website: www.MyofascialStretching.com

Email: StretchingBook@DenverMyofascialRelease.com

Credit Card: ☐ MasterCard ☐ Visa ☐ Discover	Exp. Date (mm/yy):
Account #:	
Signature:	CVC: (Last 3 #s on back of card)
Name (please print):	
Discipline:	Email:
Home Phone:	Business Phone:
Shipping Address:	Billing Address: (if different)
City:	City:
State: Zip:	State: Zip:

This form may be duplicated.

53